John McClure, (handwritten)

THANK YOU FOR
LOVING ME!

John Rice 9/23/97 (handwritten)

THE PSYCHOLOGY OF LOVING & HEALING

BY:JOHN R. RICE, M.S.W., A.C.S.W.

EDITED BY:
THOMAS J. BOTHEROYD, B.A., M.ED.
&
ZACHARY A. KNAACK, B.F.A.

PUBLISHED BY
PROFESSIONAL DEVELOPMENT, COMMUNICATION
& MARKETING CORPORATION

Published by Professional Development, Communication &
Marketing Corporation
Davie, FL.

Revised Edition
First Printing • 2,500 • January 1997

Library of Congress Card Catalog Number: 84-60233
ISBN 0-9655602-0-1

Additional copies may be obtained
by sending a check for $16.99, plus $5.00 shipping & handling; FL residents add sales tax, to the address below. For
your conveience, an order form can be found at the back of
this book.

Professional Development, Communication
& Marketing Corporation
P.O. Box 821207
South Florida, FL 33082-1207

Thank You For Loving Me may be obtained by retail outlets
at special rates. Write to the above address for information.

Printed On Recycled Paper

*M*ORRIS
PUBLISHING

3212 E. Hwy 30
Kearney, NE 68847
800-650-7888

TABLE OF CONTENTS

iii

CHAPTER IV:
DO I CHASE YOU AWAY?

CHAPTER V:
CAN I BE HELD?

CHAPTER VI:
THANK YOU FOR LOVING ME!

PREFACE

I read through the songs,
The poems,
The eloquent offerings of this book
Sitting alone late at night
Just before dawn.

These brief pieces are haunting
And beautiful to me
Because they are written so innocently,
So openly.

As I write these words,
I am taught by John Rice to say it simply
And most economically,
John Rice, You are a Beautiful Man.
You are a gift to all of us.
Thank You for You.
You teach us to LOVE.

Hugh Morgan Mill, Ph.D.
"Brother Blue"
Harvard University

MY PREMISES!

Birth,
Death,
Abuse,
Violence,
A Family Breaking Up,
Betrayal,
Desertion,
Divorce,
Separation,
Segregation,
Incarceration,

The Rejection or Fear of Rejection
By one that you love
And from whom you want the same kind
Of love and caring returned
All leave one feeling abandoned!

Abandonment,
And the fear of abandonment,
Is rejection in its highest form.

It affects each of us...
What we think of ourselves and others.
What we feel we can accept and deserve.
What we feel we can accomplish.

What we believe others think of us.
What we allow others to give us.
How well we treat ourselves and others!

The degree to which
We fear and experience abandonment,
And how we cope with these feelings,
Determines how much,
If any,
Of a corrective learning experience
Each of us will consider!

Sometimes we need to learn that an experience,
Which was to teach us, will not be the same as the
Next. And if it is, we need to look at our
Interpersonal interaction. and skills that we use
With others and learn the lesson from the
Experience.

We need to be taught first and then learn, that
Most experiences are not bad! It's that we had
A bad reaction to the experience! There is
Something to be learned from each of our
Experiences! Even death!

We need to learn how to problem solve better!
We must resolve our conflict; both internally and
externally?

History repeats itself for a reason!
Because,
We are not learning from our past
Experience!

I hope this book
Will open some doors for you
And
Encourage you to examine
And
Perhaps resolve some very painful
And
Difficult issues
It has for me!

Thank You For Loving Me and Allowing Me To Love You!

John

LOVE IS!

Love is the ultimate emotion.
To be loved,
To be able to love,
To know that I am loved,
Is the very foundation of my life!
I couldn't
And I wouldn't
Live without it!

WHY I HAVE WRITTEN THIS BOOK!

It's important to understand
How we love and choose to be loved.
It's important to understand
That sometimes if we are not loved
It's not because
We are not lovable.
It's important to understand
That sometimes we are not capable
Of really loving ourselves and others.
It's not because
We are un-loving!

Sometimes,
People that we love are simply not capable of
Giving love in return.
Sometimes
We may not feel complete
As individuals.
Perhaps
Our parents
And loved ones
Were unable to love us
The way we wanted
And needed to be loved.
Regardless of the different
Circumstances of our individual lives,
We must each learn and remember
That we are capable of both
Loving and
Being loved!

THANK YOU FOR LOVING ME!

Is a book that is written and illustrated
With feelings,
Emotions, and knowledge.

DEDICATED

To Those Who Love...
And Those Who Want To Be Loved.

CHAPTER I

I Just Discovered How Much I Love You!

What are you risking?

What are you risking?
Okay,
You risk your love!
But what else?
Are you risking your life?

That would be a sizable risk,
Wouldn't it?
There's nothing particularly dangerous
In risking your love.
You risk it
And you may lose it.

Some terrible things happen in the name
Of love.
But love is never wasted!

If we decide to take this risk together,
I may just discover how much I love you;
And, how much you love me!

It's great to know that you are loved.
To know your feelings are returned.
To know someone else is thinking of you,
Just as you're thinking of them.

Still,
I've been afraid
To tell you how much I love You.

Will I say something wrong?
Will the bubble burst?
Will I scare you away?
Will you leave me for another?

If I do accept your love,
I'll have to believe in myself
And
Accept the fact that I'm lovable!

Sounds easy?
Then,
Why does it scare me
And seem so unbelievable?

Just wait until you really know me
Before you tell me that you love me!

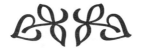

I just want to be loved!

I just want to be loved!
To be happy!
But,
I certainly don't want to suffer any pain
Because of it.
Can there be one without the other?

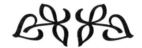

It all starts with our parents!

It all starts with our parents!
I loved you as a child
When you tossed me high above your head,
And I screamed in terror and glee.
When you let go of the seat
Of my first two wheeler,
Unknown to me!
When you always took the time to answer
My thousand and one questions,
About all those things I didn't understand.
And,
Most important,
When you tucked me in every night.
I love you even more as an adult
For now I can understand
Just how much I trusted you.
How you gave me room to grow.
How wise you were.
How much you loved me.

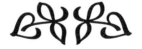

Time goes on, Life moves forward!

Time goes on, life moves forward..
Today,
We buried you Dad.
But we buried you even deeper in our hearts.
You taught us so much about life
That it hurts, and we cried.
You taught us the meaning of courage
And how to mourn the death of a loved one.
You taught us how to love and respect you,
Long after you're gone.
For you brought us together
And gave each of us something:
Ourselves and Each Other.
We stood up
And praised God for you.
Sang songs
And asked God to give us strength,
As you left our house to go to His.

We asked you to slow down,
But you couldn't;
You did what you had to do.
You were a good Man,
A good provider,
And a great teacher.

You showed us how much others loved you
As they followed behind you
Cried,
And waved good-bye
To you!

Mom!

Mom,
She completed her task here on earth.
She isn't gone.
Because She is in you,
And with you.

For your mother will live on
Through you.

You have her strength,
You have her compassion for other people.
You have her ability to care,
And reach out and touch another.

You have that place in your heart,
That sparkle in your eyes,
Just like she had when she would look
At a child.

She isn't gone;
She's with you.

Where I am!

Wherever I am,
You are!

For you are a part of me
Just as I am a part of you.

And for that,
Thank you,
And I love you!

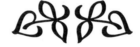

CHAPTER II

The Almighty's Image...

I need GOD in my life!

I need GOD in my life!
Not because SHE changes anything...
Not because HE fixes things up...
Not because SHE answers all my needs...
But,
Simply without THE Almighty
I wouldn't be!

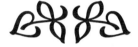

LORD, I haven't been hearing YOU!

LORD,
I haven't been hearing YOU.

Is it that YOU speak too softly for this
Noisy world?
Is it that we don't speak the same language?

Is it that I don't give YOU time,
In my busy schedule?

Or,
Could it be
That I've been too busy
Listening to myself,
To my plans,
To my hopes,
To my expectations
And all the time saying it was YOU
That I was listening to?

It is so easy to confuse ourselves with YOU,
Our voice with YOUR voice.
Need I say more?
Yes!
I'm sorry, and I Love YOU!

Thank YOU For Loving Me, LORD!

I thank YOU for today,
With its morning sun
And the refreshing coolness
Of its breeze.
For yesterday and its memories,
And for as many tomorrows
As YOU see fit
To send my way.
For each tomorrow is a gift,
A gift YOU freely give us each and every day.

Help me to see
Each of YOUR tomorrows
As something to be
Reverenced and used
As if it were to be...
The only tomorrow.

For YOU are a beautiful force,
A force we often take for granted.
YOU are the regulator of,
Yesterday, Today,
And Tomorrow.

I thank YOU for the people
That YOU have allowed to touch me.

LORD,
Allowing others to touch me
Is a risky business.
In many ways it's easier to touch others
Because
Then I'm in control.

But,
To be touched
Means to be vulnerable,
And to be vulnerable
Is a gift of YOURS
Without which
We might never allow others
Near us.

I have touched and been vulnerable;
I have learned from
And enjoyed both.
And for that gift of YOURS;
I thank YOU, and I Love YOU.

13

Some people think?

Some people think that they have to kill
To fulfill their religious beliefs.

You know...
It's *strange.*

Instead of killing
For their religious beliefs,

It's their religious beliefs
That are killing them!

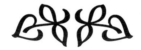

CHAPTER III

In My Image...

I had a dream!

I had a dream!
That someday I would feel no pain.
That my needs would be met,
That I would find you
And you would find me.
I had a dream...
A dream...
It's only a dream!

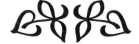

The truth is!

The truth is!
There is no perfect person
Who can make us whole.

There is no such thing as the other half;
You have to fulfill yourself.

If you are waiting
For someone to fill you up,
You will always wait in vain!
No one is equal to that task.

Waiting for another to give to you
Is only going to make you feel
Vulnerable and insecure.

One way to become
Strong,
Sure,
And whole
Is to learn how to satisfy your own needs
And, know that you can do it!

This is a very difficult lesson to learn!
It is even more difficult to stop waiting
And expecting
For someone to satisfy you.

Learn not to expect someone else
To provide for you!
Learn to provide for yourself!

Giving to yourself is the key!
Someone else can't give you,
What you won't give yourself!

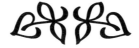

And the Search Goes On...

How easy it is to spend your life looking!

How easy it is to spend your life,
Looking for an elusive something;
Holding out for what you don't quite know.

We spend so much time looking
Without realizing...
We are only looking for ourselves.

The search for the idealized perfect other
Is always a search for what we sense
We lack.

The reason that we are never able
To find
This other person
Is that we are incapable of receiving love
As long as we feel inadequate ourselves.

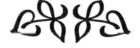

Being your friend first!

Being your friend first
Is as important
To me
As it is to you.

I want to build
A relationship with you.
Not have an affair!
I know how important it is to relate
And trust someone special.

Thank You For Loving Me!
I understand it is the foundation
That is laid now;
A foundation for a relationship
That shall stand apart
From the rest.

When I was younger!

When I was younger
I would have described love
As a physical attraction
Similar to,
But not as singular as, lust.
Gradually
It became less an activity
And more an emotion.
And just as gradually
The term lover
Became less a sexual partner,
And
More a friend.
Love and sex should certainly go together,
But
It is more important
That love and friendship do!

Sex is an action!

Sex is an action,
Not an emotion!

When the action is finished,
What's left?

You are still left with a need...
A need for friendship,
A need for someone to talk with and listen
To,
Share with,
Be with.

If that need can be filled
By your sexual partner,
That is wonderful.

But if not...
This relationship is not enough.

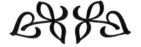

And the search goes on...

Friends are those who...

Friends are those who
Hold your hand,
Offer advice,
Give support,
Care for you.

Friend are those who give you love.
Can you possibly deny them yours?

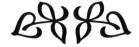

Love and friendship...

Love and friendship go together.
They both have to be worked at
To achieve something worthwhile.

But,
The benefits are certainly worth
Whatever it takes.

Love is friendship!

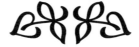

Love, what is it?

Love.
What is it?
Is love this?
Or, Is love that?
I don't know!
Devotion?
Commitment?
Infatuation?
Passion?
These emotions I know,
Are they love?

What about resentment?
Jealousy?
Dependency?

I know
That they are often mistaken
For love.

Are they love?

There is no such thing...

There is no such thing as
A love which is free
From pain and hurt.
When we accept this;
We will be able to open ourselves up;
To a freedom of emotions;
That we've never known before!

Instead of asking ourselves;
Whether there is something missing
In this relationship.
We can relax with our love.
Learn to grow with it;
And with ourselves!

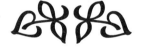

You're involved with another...

You're involved with another,
But...
I love you too!

I don't know what to do!
You see,
Someone else is fulfilling
That part of your life.
I have to respect that.

I want to see you happy.
Couldn't you be happy with me?

I will respect your present relationship,
And keep my feelings to myself!

You will never find out?

Some questions are better left unanswered!

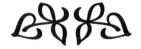

Love is!

Love is closeness.
Love is sharing.
Love is fulfillment.
Love is sacrifice.
Love is!

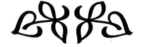

It is extremely difficult...

It is extremely difficult,
But so very important,
To accept and understand that there are no
Guarantees in life.
Nor are they in love!

There are no guarantees
That love will turn out
The way you anticipate.

There are no guarantees,
That those you love will even love you in
Return!
It's unfortunate!
There are no guaranteed rewards
In loving someone.

You can only keep working at
Loving someone
Hoping to be loved,
And finding fulfillment.

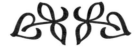

I'm sorry!

I'm sorry!
I'm not capable of hearing everything
When it is said to me.

Maybe it's because I just don't understand.
Maybe it's because I'm afraid to understand.

I have to listen to things
When I'm ready
And willing to hear them;
When I'm capable of hearing them.
I decide when I'm capable!
No one else can
Make that decision for me.
Maybe,
I just don't want to!
But,
Then again,
I must!

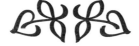

It has been said...

It has been said:
Love is a myth,
A fairy tale.

We've also said,
Falling in love,
And being in love
Are only polite euphemisms
For wanting to have sex.

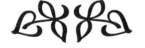

There is something...

There is something operating in each of us
That has us searching for a sexual partner.

The pressure is tremendous in itself!
But,
Additionally,
There is an urgency to cement this
Into a permanent — well,
For the time being — bonding relationship.
From going steady,
To going together...
From getting engaged
To getting married...
Only occasionally,
Is there any planning involved;
Planning of the
Financial,
Spiritual,
And
Long range
Emotional consequences.

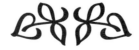

Love! For the longest time . . .

Love!
For the longest time I confused love
With emotions and feelings.
Calling the pleasant ones,
The acceptable ones love,
Harmony,
Happiness,
Joy,
Celebration,
Excitement,
Comfort,
Playfulness,
Calmness...
All of these lost their uniqueness.
Blended, became one.

But,
Anger,
Confusion,
Hurt,
Bitterness,
Loss,
Fear...

These all retained their identity
As individual emotional states.
They were never lumped into the "anti-love"
Category.

I shared with a friend...

I shared with a friend:
I'm afraid to love,
Because I was hurt before.
Getting hurt is no fun.
At first,
You wonder if
You'll ever get over it?
When you do,
You promise yourself
It will never happen again!
She said:
"You'll never find love,
If you're afraid to look!"

If you never look
And never find love,
What exactly do you have?
Nothing!

You have neither pain
Nor love.
Is a life of nothing,
What you really want?

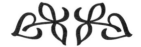

Do I prefer casual sex?

Do I prefer casual sex,
Light relationships,
Anonymous encounters?

My freedom!
What is it?

My past experiences have taught me to be
Wary of getting too close,
Too committed to another person;

And,
Not letting any one
Person
Get too close to me!
Do I want
All of the physical pleasures
I can get, without the emotional ties?

I don't just go in for one-night stands.
But,
If it begins to get more involved,
Do I try to turn it into a friendship?
And
If that isn't possible,
Would I rather cut it off completely?

It never fails
That eventually my lover discovers
That I am wonderful
And should be possessed.

Once they make that decision,
Will they never want to let go?

Do I want them to let go
Or hold on?

What do I want?

This has happened too often before.
Would I rather be lonely
And miserable;
Than go through all of that pain again?

Can I be held?

As soon as they decide that there is nobody
Better for them than me,
I get really frightened.

I panic!
I run!

Do I want to play the lovers' game?

I want to be admired,
Not clutched.
Do I really fear the complete,
Closed,
One-on-one relationship?

I can get all of the sex I want;
Without having to be involved!
So . . .
Why, should I bother with all of the
Emotional,
Spiritual, and
Intellectual attachments?

I don't know what I am afraid of!
I think,
Perhaps,
It is of things that I don't understand!

Am I afraid of a commitment?
Am I not afraid of being alone...
Only of being rejected?

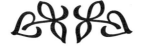

It is one of the greatest ironies...

It is one of the greatest ironies of love,
That the emotion
Which brings you
The greatest pleasure
And fulfillment;
Should also be capable,
Of
Bringing you,
The greatest pain and emptiness.

I have learned...

I have learned,
That to demonstrate anger honestly;
To say what is bothering me about
A specific incident that happened between us;
Without name calling and false accusations;
Can be as high of an expression of love,
As the gentlest gesture.

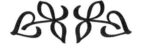

Emotions and feelings...

Emotions and feelings,
Are like faces that love wears.

Actions and deeds,
Are the real expression
Of love !

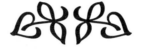

Can you understand?

Can you understand,
How someone may OD?
Can you understand,
How someone would want to end their
Existence?

Can you understand,
Why someone would never want to sober up?
Can you understand,
Why someone would never want to come down?
Can you understand,
Why someone would want to love everyone?
Can you understand,
Why someone wouldn't want to be involved with
Anyone?

Can you understand?

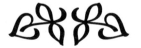

If you haven't experienced!

If you haven't experienced what I'm talking about,
Then,
You really don't understand, what I'm talking
About!

You may have heard about it!
You may have talked about it!
You may have read about it!
But,
You still don't understand, because you
Haven't experienced it, the way I have!

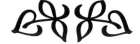

And the search goes on...

Where does love begin?

Where does love begin?
How does it start?
It is a warm sensation that flows
Through your body?
Or,
Is it a flash that jolts you?
Love starts from an initial,
Unexplainable attraction;
Commonly referred to as infatuation.
This infatuation isn't love!
Only the first steps, in a process
Towards a full involvement of caring
And understanding.
But, it is essential!
Without it,
Love can never develop and grow.
Isn't there a cliché about love being
Like a fine wine?
Age and time will refine the mixture,
But, the grapes have to be just right
At the start,
For something special to develop!

There are two stages...

There are two stages of love:
The first is that crazy love,
That just zaps you after
The initial meeting.

Then that deep,
Meaningful love that develops,
As you become more comfortable
And familiar.

These feelings are worlds apart!

The first kind of love,
Sends you soaring into the clouds!
You are walking on air,
Nothing bothers you!
Except the person you love.

Your waking moments are dreamlike.
It is as if you are in a trance...
And you are!

You're in love!

Eventually,
You may awaken from this trance,
Into the second kind of love.
This second kind of love takes longer!
It comes from knowing someone very
Closely,
Becoming intimate and
Familiar with all parts of their life.

It comes from trust,
Feeling at ease,
Being concerned and
Caring.

It is a relaxed and comfortable feeling.
It is not as uplifting
And heavy,
As the first kind or love.
But,
Far more rewarding in its' security.
But, not as easy to obtain.

CHAPTER IV

Do I Chase You Away?

What do you want?

What do you want?

What do you want from me?
What are you looking for?
Are you looking for someone to love
You?

If you're looking for a lover,
Look for someone who is also a friend.

The ideal lover is a friend who loves!

Whenever I see someone...

Whenever I see someone I like,
I always assume that they are taken!

Should I assume?

Is it possible that my assuming,
Is just a protection I've mastered;
To avoid,
Taking the risk of not assuming?

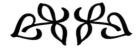

I met someone...

I met someone yesterday!

A person whose smile was contagious;

And

Whose voice was so inviting!

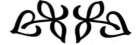

If I were?

If I were honest
And opened myself up to you.
Told you exactly what was on my mind.
Would you still be my friend?
Would you be frightened off?
Keep your distance!
Turn your back on me?
Perhaps you are frightened
For the same reasons.

Can I be honest with you?

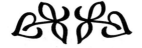

I wonder?

I wonder
What would it be like?
If I knew myself,
Like others do?
I'm so close to myself,
That I miss a lot!
It's like looking into the mirror.
I never see every angle of myself,
At least,
Not like the person standing next to me.
What if I could see every angle?
Would I want to?

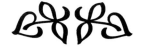

Would I chase you?

Would I chase you away,
By telling you what my needs are?
Could these needs that we are afraid to
Share,
Actually be helping us
To grow within each other?
In dealing with each other's needs,
Do we really get what we need from
Each other?

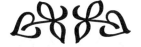

What should I do?

What should I do?
When I'm in a power struggle with someone
I love?

I could give in
So one of us could be happy!
But,
What about my integrity?
My principles?
Do I say "quits,"
And have both of us lose?

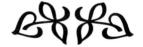

Before we can talk!

Before we can talk about meeting
Each other's needs;
I have to first know
What my needs are!
And,
That isn't easy!

Needs have a strange way of changing.
What I thought I needed today is often
Forgotten by tomorrow.

And what about you?
Are you any different?
Is it any easier for you;
To know what you need?

> *Am I ready*
> *And*
> *Willing to meet my needs?*

> *Are you ready*
> *And*
> *Willing to meet your needs?*

Only after we hare answered these questions
Can each of us ask:

Am I ready and willing to meet your needs?
Are you ready and willing to to meet mine?

You said that?

You said that before?
You even remember when and where you said it!

Where was I?
You know,
Just because I wasn't listening,
I never knew!

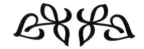

And The Search Goes On...

I finally fell...

I finally fell in love;
I thought this day would never come.
I have someone who is in love with me!

Nothing can compare
With this feeling of being loved.
With someone who
Is in love with me!

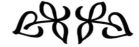

I'm sorry!

I'm sorry!
I have never demanded
So much from anyone.

I have never asked
So much from anyone.

I'm sorry!
But it is because,
I have never loved anyone
Like you!

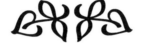

I'm not sorry that I...

I'm not sorry that I said it!
Same things just need to be said!

Let's resolve it;
So we can go on.

I love you !

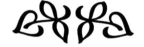

There are times when...

There are times when saying:
I love you!
Is just not enough.

It's not enough to take away the pain.
It's not enough to explain.
Or,
Make things clearer.

It's just not enough!

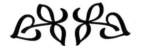

When I am silent...

When I'm silent,
It's not always because I have nothing to
say!
It's just that I am afraid to say it!

You see I have much to say,
Questions to ask,
Observations to make.

Sometimes,
When I'm silent,
It's
Because,
I'm not sure
If I can cope
With how you may answer my questions.
Or,
What you might say about my observations.

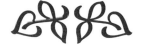

Wow!

Wow!
How come we haven't had this conversation
Before?

No!
Wait!
Don't answer that!

I just figured it out.
I wasn't ready for it!

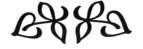

You know!

You know!
You really feel good!
I really feel good!

Better yet,
We really feel good together!

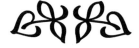

At times I feel...

At times I feel
So intensely
It surprises me.

They are my feelings!
No one else can imagine
How much they affect me.

How much joy
Or,
Pain they cause.

Isn't it strange?
How easy it is to forget.

That,
I am not
The only one to feel!

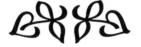

If we would only be...

If we would only be more aware of what
We are doing to others.
How we touch them.
Not only with our hands,
But by just being there.

We need to be aware of the effects our
Presence is having on others.
As it is happening!

If we would,
People could be more together!
In a refreshing,
Caring way.
If we would care what we are doing to others!

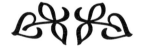

I don't want to be in love..

I don't want to be in love with you.
I don't want to want and be afraid to ask.
I don't want and want and have to ask.
I don't want to want and not receive.

In other words,
I don't want to want.

But,
That's life!

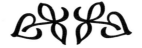

Thank You For Loving Me!

CHAPTER V

Can I Be Held?

It was a moment...

It was a moment of craziness!
Thank GOD,
I saw that!
For I thought,
If it wasn't for the pain that I would
Leave with you and others;
I would not be existing today.

But, why was that?
Was I feeling lonely and helpless?
And,
Not capable of getting my needs met?

Was I angry that you didn't choose
To meet them?

You see,
Love is my strongest need!
At times, I am so infantile that
When you are not around me
I'm like a newborn child,
Who thinks his mother has abandoned him;
And cries each time
He loses sight of her.

Am I substituting this new love
For the love of a parent
Who has abandoned me?

We all experience
Abandonment at birth.

When our parents cannot raise us,
We all experience a void in our lives.
A need to find our origin,
Identity,
And ask,
Why have you abandoned me?

Am I not good enough?

Do you not love and want me?

You see,

If I think you don't love me,

Then I cannot accept

Someone else loving me!

What right have I to ask you for more than
You are giving me now?

You're beautiful,
So beautiful!
That even the blind can see;
When they are near you.

The deaf can hear;
When you stand still.

That is why
So many people love you.

At times I feel
I'm just another mouth for you to feed.
Another person to support and comfort.

This is me talking!
Can I listen?
And, learn to limit?
And, take
Responsibility
For my needs?

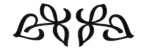

When I say no...

When I say No sometimes,
It's really myself I'm saying No to!

I'm not saying NO to you.
I'm not rejecting you.
I'm rejecting me!

But,
How could you know that?

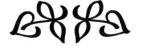

Have you noticed?

Have you noticed?
That, I haven't been
Around much lately?

I'm not staying away from you
Because, I don't love you!

Sometimes the greatest love
Demands some time and space.

It isn't that I'm staying away from you
Because, I don't love you.
It's because I do !

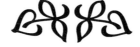

Was my love?

Was my love self-centered?
When I was "in love",
I was loving only my image of who
And what I was seeing.

You were not allowed to be yourself.
I had no concern for your needs.
I cared only about an image.
I had placed you on a pedestal.
Totally ignoring how destructive that
Position was for you and for me.

If we discover...

If we discover that we no longer
Love each other the same way.
Don't try to persuade yourself
That, I didn't love you!
Don't!

You are still important to me.
Do you hear that?
I cannot love you,
And want you
The same way
That you love and want me.

I feel very strongly
That I never can again.
I don't want to live the rest of my
Life this way!
And, I'm sure
That you don't want to either.

It isn't something that either of us
Has done.
Or,
Not done.
It isn't something that can be corrected
Or ignored.

I need to think about myself now,
And
Find out what makes me happy.

I can't do this with you.
I can't do this with anyone right now.
I must do this alone.

I would go to great lengths
To keep from hurting you,
But,
I can only do that up to a certain point.
The point at which I would be hurting myself.

I have thought
And thought
About all of this.
Still,
I always come back to the same answer.

We would not be happy together.
Yes,
This makes me almost unbearably sad.
But
I must be fair to you,
And honest with myself!

I'm loved by...

I'm loved by,
And have become involved with another!
What do I tell you?

Do I ask you to please forgive me
And keep your distance
And try not to become involved with me?
Do I just let things go along
Without explaining
And leave you to deal with it as best you
can?

What if I become cold and distant?
Would you think that I just don't care?
Would you think I'm playing hard to get?
Would you think I'm afraid and running?
Would you think I'm abandoning you?

Is it better to just be honest
And say that I have found someone else?
That I'm loved by another!

I'm sorry I'm not capable...

I'm sorry!
I'm not capable of understanding
And accepting what you are offering me
Right now.
Perhaps I never will.

I'm sorry for the pain that I see
In your eyes,
Because,
I feel that pain in my heart.

I ask that you forgive me,
But,
I understand why you probably can't

At least not now!

81

Thank You For Loving Me!

CHAPTER VI

Thank You For Loving Me!

Thank You For...

Thank You For Loving Me!
For,
I'm writing about you
And,
I'm writing about me.

If anything had been different,
We could not have shared
This time together.

And, I love you!

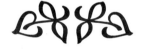

I love you!

I love you!
I cherish your friendship,
Your love,
Your respect.
The thought of you
Make. me warm and secure inside.
Time has only confirmed my feelings.
As my love for you has only grown.
I now realize how much
A part of my life you have been.
You have partly shaped my personality
And my being.

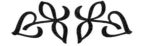

Thank You For Loving Me!

The key to peace is...

The key to peace
Is to assist each of us to
Feel,
And be secure
Within ourselves!
And,
Until we can;
We
Will not be able to respect each other!
Because,
We will not be able
To respect OURSELVES!

Understand this!
That, in order for me to respect myself,
I have to love myself!
RESPECT OF ONESELF IS LOVE!
And,
Without loving myself,
I am not capable of loving
And, caring about you!

And, you abusing me,
Hating me and raping me!
Bombing me,
Destroying me and my sense of well-being.
Denying me the same rights and privileges
That you enjoy.
These actions don't make me respect you
Or fear you!
They make me hate you
And hate me!
I can't respect you;
When you don't respect me!

And,
Without me loving me,
And me loving you!

And you loving you;
And, you loving me!

There cannot be any lasting PEACE!

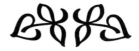

Thank you. . . It hasn't been easy. . .

Thank You For Loving Me!

It hasn't been easy discovering love,

Even though it has been around me since Birth .

You know,

We don't always know what we have!

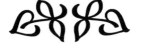

Thank you...for teaching...

Thank You For Loving Me!

It hasn't been easy understanding love.

Thank you for teaching me about it!

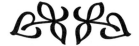

Thank you . . . Because . . .

Thank You For Loving Me!

It hasn't been easy to accept love,

Because I haven't always known

That love was mine to accept.

And,

Once I did know it,

I wasn't sure what to do with it.

Now I do!

I can love;

And let myself be loved!

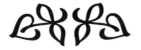

Thank you...I have experienced!

Thank you for loving me!

I have experienced feelings

And gained knowledge that I would

Never have known

If it weren't for you!

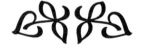

Thank you . . . You know!

Thank You For Loving Me!

For you have given me the wisdom

And the courage to be all that I can be!

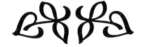

Thank You For Loving Me!

Thank You For Loving Me!
You Know Who You Are!
I Know Who I Am!

We Now Know,
Love and Respect,
Ourselves & Each Other!

The End!

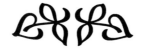

EPILOGUE

I ask each of you who read this book or listen to its words to continue to make a difference in your life and of those around you. You are capable of loving yourself and others. You need to identify and heal your own unresolved abandonment issues. It takes a strong individual to look at himself or herself and ask, how can I improve on myself so I can be a better person and communicate with others more effectively?

You must help your children, family members, friends and neighbors to do the same. You must avoid judging others. Encourage each person. Assist them to grow-up and develop a positive attitude about themselves and life. Don't react to situations, problem solve!

In order for us to live together as the one (1) race of Human Beings that we are, we must love and respect ourselves and each others! You must feel secure and not be threatened by people that are different from yourself.

You must be accepting of all skin colors, nationalities, religious beliefs, sexual preferences, genders and languages of the Human Race.

None of us is better than the other!

If we believe we are better than others, we are too self-centered and insecure. You see, if we really feel good about ourselves, people of different cultures would not threaten us!

Understand that history is repeating itself for a reason! History is not in control of the Human Race and recycling our experiences according to a history clock! The Human Race is in control of its' history!

History is not repeating its' behaviors and mistakes, Humans are! We have not learned our lessons!

95

History has shown us that each time we hated our neighbors we destroyed them and ourselves!

History has shown us that when we didn't care what was happening to our neighbors, the same events happened to us!

History has shown us that when we don't resolve conflicts and forgive people and their governments for their wrong doings, Humans are the only ones to die and be buried!

You can look around the world and see all of the ethnic and religious wars that are threatening to kill Humanity!

Some groups feel that their group should be the only group of people!

Some groups feel that only their religious beliefs should exist!

They are both wrong!

These thoughts and behaviors are selfish, childish and insecure!

As I said in my book, "You know it's strange that people feel they have to kill for their religious beliefs. You know it's strange, instead of killing for their religious beliefs; it's their religious beliefs that are killing them!"

There is pathology in every society and religion. Human Beings have written this into our history! Not your GOD! Your GOD is present in your life to give you guidance in living a better life; strength to problem solve and cope with life's experience; to have peace now and forever and to give praise to a higher power!

We must begin to look at everyday events, behaviors, issues and reactions as expressions of how well we are caring for people. You must understand that our thoughts and actions are causing the destruction of people and societies.

Look at how child, sexual, physical and emotional abuse damage people and cause them to act out at love ones and society. We must continue to facilitate corrective learning experiences in individuals and in society! We must stop destroying poeple, because they will just destroy us in return!

We must accept the differences in each other and build upon our strengths and common needs! You have the same rights as everyone else! If your rights are denied, my rights are not secured!

We must stop the killing fields in our homes, streets, communities and nations of the world.

We must stop entertaining ourselves with bloodshed and violence!

We must stop being selfish in our behaviors and actions!

Understanding that we keep destroying our children, mates, families, communities, and nations because we haven't addressed the issues that all of us have in common! Unresolved issues of abandonment, caused by our lack of caring, concern, acceptance, understanding and greed!

We are producing children and adults that have a damaged sense of pride and self-worth.

Some feel that they have nothing to live for!

Others feel they have reasons to die for!

Both are incorrect!

You can't raise the children of the world without caring for them!

You can't be safe, if others are not!

History is repeating itself because only the people are dying, not the conflicts and our pain. This is why we must resolve abandonment issues and provide corrective learning experiences that teach people how to love themselves and others.

"Please! Let the people live and let the conflicts die!"

Thank You For Loving Me!
John

ABOUT THE AUTHOR

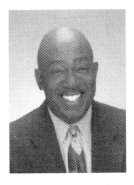

John R. Rice, is a professional speaker, trainer and Certified Professional Consultant. As a Social Worker, he has been recognized for his contributions to society in, "Who Who's In The World."

He is Chairman of the Board for Professional Development, Communication and Marketing Corporation in Davie, Florida.

Their mission is to provide you with training, services and products that improves the quality of your life and business. If they can be of service to you, your business or organization, please contact them at (954) 4̶3̶4̶-̶6̶8̶2̶1̶.

Their website on the Internet is: *680 - 4867*
http://johnrice.com

Email - solution @ icanect. net

To order books by mail, send $16.99, plus $5.00 for postage and handling, per copy to:

P.O. Box 821207 • South Florida, FL 33082-1207

Florida residents, please add 6% sales tax, plus discretionary surtax if applicable.

To book John Rice as a keynote speaker, please contact The American Speakers Bureau Corporation in Orlando, Florida. (407) 826-4248.

To order additional copies of **Thank You For Loving Me! The Psychology of Loving & Healing**, complete the information below.

Ship to: (please print)

Name _____

Address _____

City, State, Zip _____

Day phone _____

_____ copies of *Thank You* @ $16.99 each $ _____

Postage and handling @ $5.00 per book $ _____

FL residents add 6% tax $ _____

Total amount enclosed $ _____

Make checks payable to *Professional Development, Communication & Marketing Corporation*

Send to: P.O. Box 821207
South FL, FL 33082-1207

- -

To order additional copies of **Thank You For Loving Me! The Psychology of Loving & Healing**, complete the information below.

Ship to: (please print)

Name _____

Address _____

City, State, Zip _____

Day phone _____

_____ copies of *Thank You* @ $16.99 each $ _____

Postage and handling @ $5.00 per book $ _____

FL residents add 6% tax $ _____

Total amount enclosed $ _____

Make checks payable to *Professional Development, Communication & Marketing Corporation*

Send to: P.O. Box 821207
South FL, FL 33082-1207